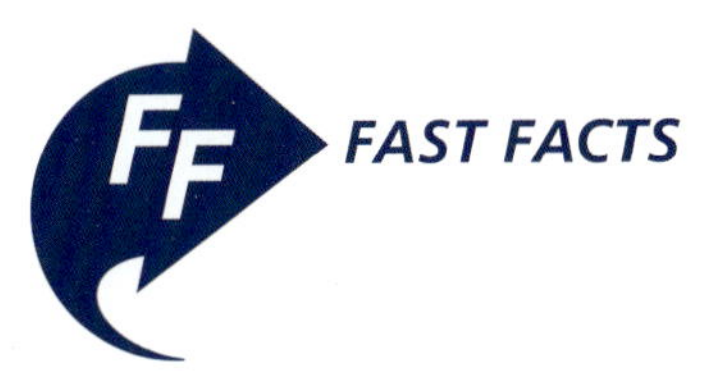

Recognizing Refractory Myasthenia Gravis

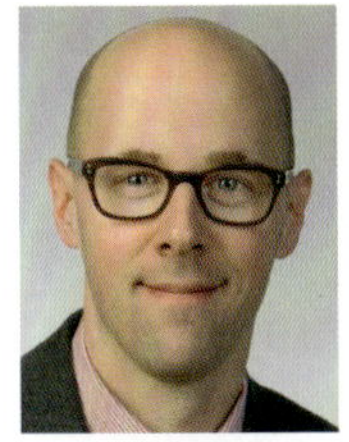

Nicholas J Silvestri MD
Clinical Associate Professor of Neurology
University at Buffalo Jacobs School of
Medicine and Biomedical Sciences
Department of Neurology
Buffalo General Hospital
Buffalo, NY, USA

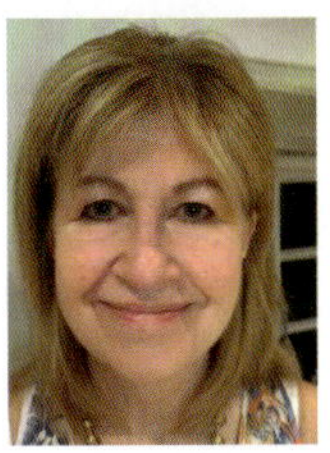

Jacqueline A Palace MD
Consultant Neurologist
Nuffield Department of Clinical Neurosciences
John Radcliffe Hospital
Oxford, UK

Declaration of Independence
This book is as balanced and as practical as we can make it.
Ideas for improvement are always welcome at **fastfacts.com**

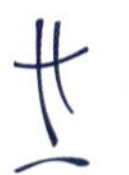
HEALTH PRESS

Fast Facts: Recognizing Refractory Myasthenia Gravis
First published March 2018

Health Press Limited, Elizabeth House, Queen Street, Abingdon, Oxford OX14 3LN, UK
Tel: +44 (0)1235 523233

Book orders can be placed by telephone or via the website.
To order via the website, please go to: fastfacts.com
For telephone orders, please call +44 (0)1752 202301

A CIP record for this title is available from the British Library.

ISBN 978-1-910797-53-2

Silvestri N (Nicholas)
Fast Facts: Recognizing Refractory Myasthenia Gravis/
Nicholas J Silvestri, Jacqueline A Palace

Cover illustration: light micrograph showing motor nerve endings; iron hemotoylin stain 126× by Alvin Telser, Science Photo Library
Medical illustrations by Graeme Chambers.
Typesetting by Thomas Bohm, User Design, Illustration and Typesetting, UK.
Printed in the UK with Xpedient Print.

An independent publication developed by Health Press Limited and provided as a service to medicine. Supported by Alexion®.

Alexion®, and many other stakeholders, received the opportunity to review the manuscript prior to publication. Full editorial control was retained by the authors and Health Press Limited.

GL/UNB-gMG/17/0026
US/UNB-gMG/17/0056

Glossary 4

Introduction 5

Definition and epidemiology 7

Pathophysiology and classification 13

Diagnosis and management: an overview 23

Assessment of disease severity and treatment response 32

Useful resources 44

Index 45

Glossary

Acetylcholine receptor (AChR) antibody: pathogenic antibody that causes complement-mediated destruction, direct blockade and/or increased internalization of AChRs.

Complement: portion of the immune system that enhances the activity of antibodies in removing pathogens, predominantly by attacking the pathogen's membrane, and promotes the inflammatory response.

Fatigability: fluctuating weakness; typically, symptoms worsen with prolonged physical activity or as the day goes on.

Generalized myasthenia gravis (MG): MG with diffuse involvement of muscles beyond just the ocular muscles.

Juvenile myasthenia gravis: MG with disease onset before 18 years of age.

Muscle receptor tyrosine kinase (MuSK) antibody: pathogenic antibody in a minority of patients with generalized MG, with a distinct phenotype.

Myasthenia gravis: most common disorder of the neuromuscular junction; a classic autoimmune disease that is most commonly caused by antibodies to the AChR and less frequently to MuSK.

Myasthenic crisis: respiratory failure or severe bulbar dysfunction caused by MG, necessitating intubation and mechanical ventilation until clinical improvement in strength occurs.

Neuromuscular junction: a synapse between a motor neuron terminal and the folded endplate membrane, a highly excitable region of the muscle fiber where action potentials are initiated across the muscle surface.

Ocular myasthenia gravis: MG with involvement of ocular muscles only; typically manifests as ptosis, diplopia or difficulty with eye closure.

Refractory myasthenia gravis: a subset of patients with MG who have inadequate responses to appropriate immunosuppressive therapy.

Repetitive nerve stimulation: a specialized nerve conduction study often used in the diagnosis of MG; electrodecrement indicates a disorder of neuromuscular transmission.

Seronegative myasthenia gravis: the term applied to patients with MG in whom AChR or MuSK antibodies are not detected, and patients diagnosed with MG by clinical or electrodiagnostic means.

Single fiber electromyography: a specialized form of electromyography with a high sensitivity in diagnosing disorders of the neuromuscular junction such as MG.

Thymoma: tumor of the thymus.

Thymus: a specialized primary lymphoid organ of the immune system located in the superior mediastinum and frequently involved in the pathogenesis of MG.

Introduction

Myasthenia gravis (MG) is the most common disorder of the neuromuscular junction. It is a classic autoimmune disease, characterized by muscle 'fatigability', most commonly caused by antibodies to the acetylcholine receptor (AChR) and less frequently to muscle receptor tyrosine kinase (MuSK).

The presentation of MG in any given patient is variable. Approximately two-thirds of patients initially present with ocular symptoms, including ptosis and diplopia, but the disease becomes generalized (i.e. it spreads beyond the eye muscles) in over 80% of patients. These patients have a predilection for bulbar, facial, neck and proximal limb muscle involvement. The muscles of respiration may also be affected, leading to dyspnea on exertion or orthopnea.

Most patients with MG are able to live productive lives with few or no symptoms when adequately treated. A distinct subset of patients, however, have very difficult-to-control disease. These patients, who continue to have symptoms because of an inadequate response to appropriate immunosuppressive therapy, are often referred to as having refractory or treatment-refractory MG.

Here, we examine how this subset of patients presents, and the assessment tools to use to set a benchmark by which patients' progress can be monitored in order to identify individuals who are no longer responding to treatment. Recognizing this subset of patients is essential, as newer treatment strategies are beginning to emerge that may be effective in this group.

This resource is of value to neurologists, neurology trainees and ophthalmologists caring for patients with MG; indeed, all clinicians with an interest in this rare disease. Patients who wish to know more and have a deeper dialog with their doctor or patient group may also find this text just what they are looking for.

1 Definition and epidemiology

Definition of treatment-refractory myasthenia gravis

There is no standard definition of refractory myasthenia gravis (MG), but studies have generally utilized the criteria shown in Table 1.1.

Prevalence and incidence

Several epidemiological studies examining the incidence and prevalence of generalized MG have been performed worldwide over the past few decades, most of which have been conducted in Europe. These studies have reported a wide range in incidence rates (IR) and prevalence rates (PR). In a large meta-analysis, the estimated IR was 5.3 per million person-years with a range of 1.7 to 21.3.[3] In another systematic review, the most reliable IR was 30 per one million per year.[4] The prevalence rate has been found to be 77.67 cases per million, and a range of 15–179 per million worldwide has been reported.[3]

Both IR and PR have been shown to be increasing over time in a non-linear fashion, with both IR and PR roughly doubling around 1980.[3] This is most likely attributable to greater awareness and accurate diagnosis of the disease, improvements in diagnostic testing

TABLE 1.1

Criteria used to define treatment-refractory myasthenia gravis[1,2]

- Fails to respond to otherwise adequate doses and durations of conventional immunosuppressive treatments
- Requires excessive amounts of potentially harmful agents
- Requires repeated rescue treatment with short-term therapies such as intravenous immunoglobulin and plasma exchange
- Frequent myasthenic crises
- Unacceptable adverse reactions to conventional treatments and/or comorbidities that preclude the use of conventional treatments

(e.g. antibody testing), epidemiological methodology and more effective treatment of the disorder, leading to better long-term survival.

When adequately treated, most patients with MG are able to live productive lives with few or no symptoms. A distinct subset of patients, however, have very aggressive and difficult-to-control disease. These patients, who continue to have symptoms and are at continuing risk of crisis and exacerbation because of an inadequate response to appropriate immunosuppressive therapy, are often referred to as having treatment-refractory MG. The exact prevalence of refractory myasthenia is unknown, but it is estimated to occur in approximately 10–15% of patients with generalized disease.[2,5]

In a large retrospective study by Suh et al. of 128 sequential patients seen in a large tertiary referral center, 19 (14.8%) patients were found to be treatment-refractory.[5] The definition of refractory included those patients who could not lower their immunotherapy without clinical relapse, were not clinically controlled on their immunotherapy regimen, or experienced severe side effects from immunotherapy. This study may have overestimated the true incidence of refractory MG as it was conducted at a large tertiary clinic, where the referral population comprised patients with more active disease.

In a recent study by Sudulagunta et al., 76 of 512 patients (14.8%) in referral centers in India were classified as having refractory MG[6] – exactly the same incidence as in the study discussed above.

Age and sex

The incidence of generalized MG has been found to have a bimodal age distribution, with a peak around 30 years of age and again at 50 years, with a steady rise in incidence thereafter. Female cases predominate in the younger age group and males in the older (Figure 1.1).[3,7] Juvenile MG is defined as disease with onset before the age of 18 years and accounts for roughly 10% of all cases of MG.[7]

In the Suh et al. study discussed above, the median age of the refractory group was 36 years versus 60 years in the non-refractory group. Refractory patients were more likely to be female (14 of 19).[5] In the Sudulagunta et al. study, the age of disease onset in the refractory MG group was significantly lower than in the non-refractory group (median age of 36 years versus 61 years). The refractory group also had a higher percentage of females.[6]

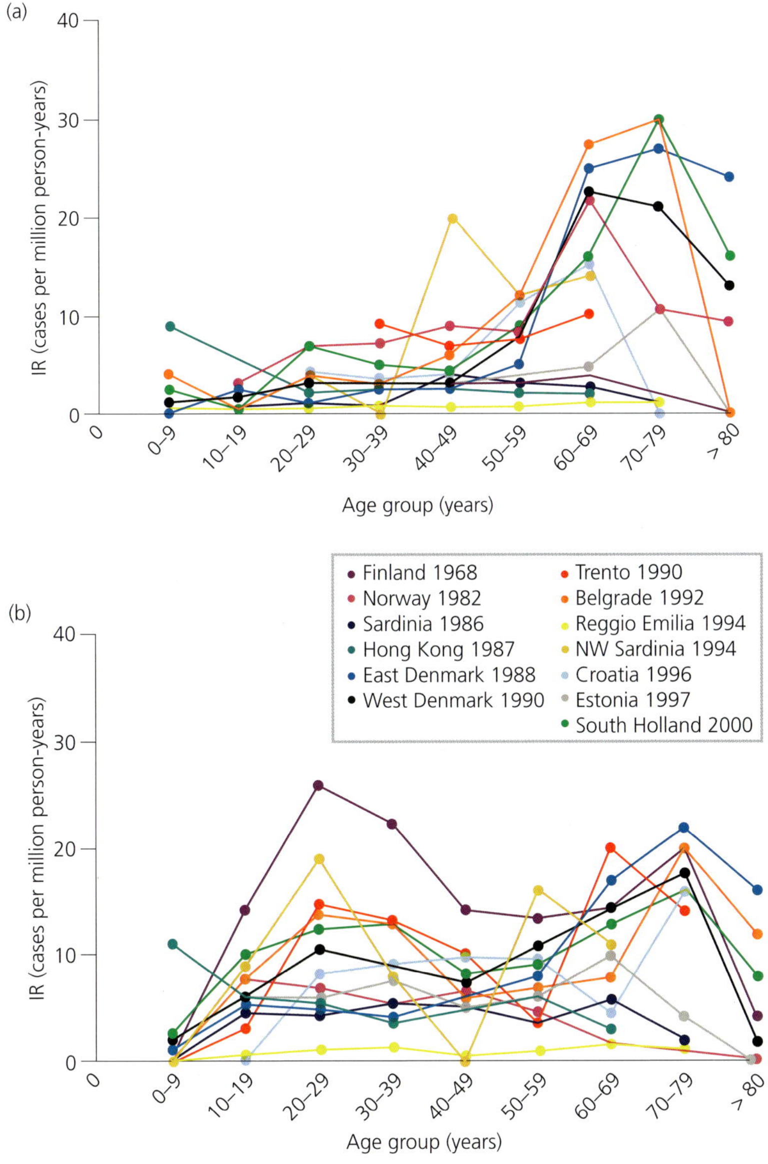

Figure 1.1 Age-specific incidence rates of myasthenia gravis in (a) males and (b) females. Overall, all populations show an increase in the frequency of disease with age. Reproduced with permission from Carr AS et al. 2010, under a Creative Commons Attribution License.[3]

Geography and ethnicity

In general, MG is more commonly reported in East Asia, with a higher frequency of ocular disease.[8,9] There is otherwise an equal geographic distribution in the incidence and prevalence of MG in both adults and children.

While all races and ethnicities are affected by MG, people of African descent have a slightly higher prevalence of the disease, which is particularly true in muscle receptor tyrosine kinase (MuSK) antibody-positive disease.[7,10] MuSK antibody-positive disease is also more commonly reported in geographic locations closer to the equator.[11]

Genetics. There may be a hereditary predisposition to develop MG as there is an increased incidence of certain HLA antigens including HLA-B8, HLA-DRw3, and HLA-DQw2 in various MG populations.[12]

MuSK-antibody positivity and other clinical characteristics

Suh et al. found that 47% of treatment-refractory patients were MuSK-antibody positive, compared with 2% of non-refractory patients.[5] Despite the high percentage of patients with MuSK antibodies in the refractory group, they were also more likely to have undergone thymectomy and to have had thymoma.[5]

Sudulagunta et al. found that 36 (47.36%) of the refractory patients had MuSK antibodies. Patients in the refractory group were also more likely to have thymoma, diabetes mellitus and dyslipidemia.[6] The high incidence of diabetes and dyslipidemia was thought to be secondary to the higher doses of corticosteroids used in the refractory group and highlights some of the risks associated with long-term corticosteroid treatment.

Key points – definition and epidemiology

- Treatment-refractory MG is defined as disease that inadequately responds, or results in unacceptable adverse reactions, to conventional immunosuppressive treatments, or requires excessive amounts of potentially harmful agents or repeated rescue therapy.
- Patients with comorbidities that preclude the use of conventional treatments and/or who have frequent myasthenic crises are also considered to have refractory MG.
- Treatment-refractory myasthenia gravis (MG) is estimated to occur in approximately 10–15% of patients with generalized MG.
- Compared with non-refractory patients, treatment-refractory patients are more likely to be younger at disease onset, female, thymomatous and muscle receptor tyrosine kinase (MuSK)-antibody positive.

References

1. Drachman DB, Adams RN, Hu R et al. Rebooting the immune system with high-dose cyclophosphamide for treatment of refractory myasthenia gravis. *Ann N Y Acad Sci* 2008;1132:305–14.

2. Silvestri NJ, Wolfe GI. Treatment-refractory myasthenia gravis. *J Clin Neuromuscul Dis* 2014;15:167–78.

3. Carr AS, Cardwell CR, McCarron PO, McConville J. A systematic review of population based epidemiological studies in myasthenia gravis. *BMC Neurol* 2010;10:46.

4. McGrogan A, Sneddon S, deVries CS. The incidence of myasthenia gravis: a systematic literature review. *Neuroepidemiology* 2010;34:171–83.

5. Suh J, Goldstein JM, Nowak RJ. Clinical characteristics of refractory myasthenia gravis patients. *Yale J Biol Med* 2013;86:255–60.

6. Sudulagunta SR, Sepehrar M, Sodalagunta MB et al. Refractory myasthenia gravis – clinical profile, comorbidities and response to rituximab. *Ger Med Sci* 2016;14:1–15.

7. Phillips LH 2nd, Torner JC, Anderson GS, Cox GM. The epidemiology of myasthenia gravis in central and western Virginia. *Neurology* 1992;42:1888–93.

8. Yu YL, Hawkins BR, Ip MS et al. Myasthenia gravis in Hong Kong Chinese. 1. Epidemiology and adult disease. *Acta Neurol Scand* 1992;86:113–19.

9. Lok W et al. Myasthenia gravis in Singapore. *Neurol J Southeast Asia* 2003;8:35–40.

10. Oh SJ, Morgan MB, Lu L et al. Racial differences in myasthenia gravis in Alabama. *Muscle Nerve* 2009;39:328–32.

11. Vincent A. Autoantibodies in neuromuscular transmission disorders. *Ann Indian Acad Neurol* 2008;11:140–5.

12. Meriggioli MN, Sanders DB. Autoimmune myasthenia gravis: emerging clinical and biological heterogeneity. *Lancet Neurol* 2009;8:475–90.

Further reading

Deymeer F, Gungor-Tuncer O, Yilmaz V et al. Clinical comparison of anti-MuSK- vs anti-AChR-positive and seronegative myasthenia gravis. *Neurology* 2007;68:609–11.

Grob D, Brunner N, Namba T, Pagala M. Lifetime course of myasthenia gravis. *Muscle Nerve* 2008;37:141–9.

Phillips LH 2nd. The epidemiology of myasthenia gravis. *Ann N Y Acad Sci* 2003;998:407–12.

Phillips LH 2nd, Torner JC. Epidemiologic evidence for a changing natural history of myasthenia gravis. *Neurology* 1996;47:1233–8.

2 Pathophysiology and classification

Normal neuromuscular transmission

At the normal neuromuscular junction (NMJ), acetylcholine (ACh) is released from the motor neuron terminal, diffuses across the synaptic space and binds to ACh receptors (AChR), which are densely clustered on the folded endplate membrane of the muscle fiber. The high concentration of AChRs is crucial for efficient neuromuscular transmission. The ACh depolarizes the muscle endplate region, ultimately causing the muscle to contract (Figure 2.1).

Pathophysiology

Myasthenia gravis (MG) is the best characterized autoimmune disorder of the nervous system. The immune-mediated nature of MG was suspected as early as the 1960s when it was speculated to be caused by a dysregulated immune response, with antibodies directed against skeletal muscle.[1]

Acetylcholine receptor antibodies. A series of animal and human experiments in the 1970s confirmed the above hypothesis, and elevated titers of antibodies against the acetylcholine receptor (AChR) were ultimately discovered in the serum of patients with MG.[2] Loss of AChRs results in impaired neuromuscular transmission and muscle weakness.

Multiple pathological processes cause loss of functional AChRs in MG:

- complement-mediated lysis
- accelerated internalization and degradation of AChRs
- direct blockade of AChRs by antibodies.[3,4]

Complement-mediated lysis is thought to be the most important mode of loss of AChR, but the actual process that initiates the aberrant immune attack on the AChR is unknown. Both the immunoglobulin (Ig) G antibody and complement have been localized to the motor endplate in myasthenia models, indicating that circulating IgG antibodies directed against the AChR bind to the postsynaptic membrane and activate the terminal complement sequence (C5b–9),

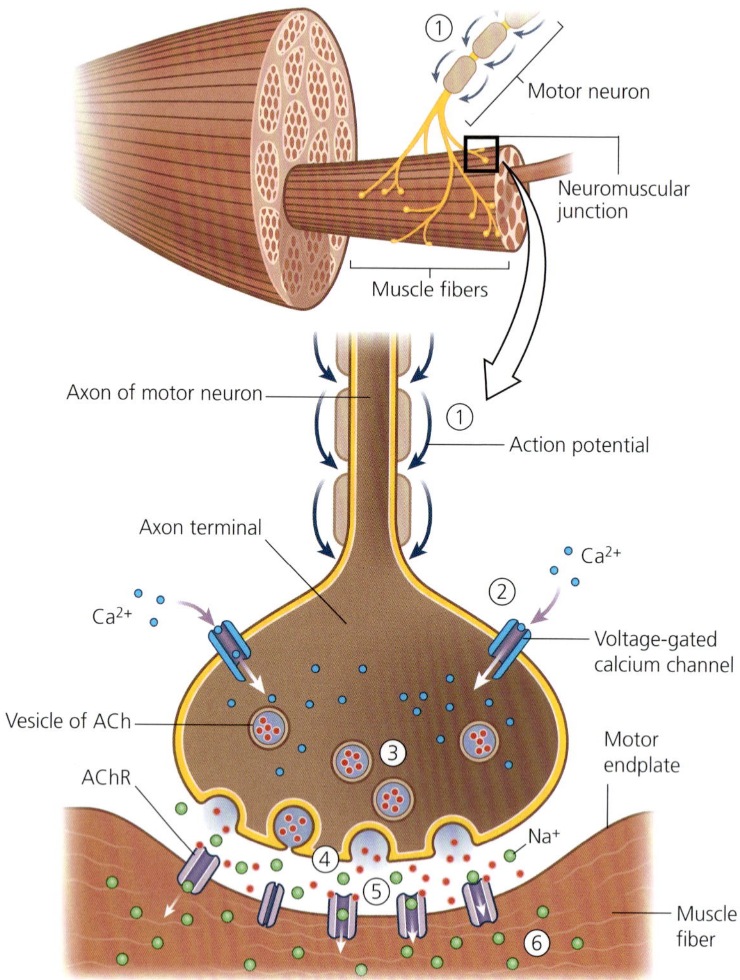

Figure 2.1 A single motor neuron can stimulate several muscle fibers. At the neuromuscular junction: (1) an action potential spreads over the motor neuron terminal, (2) opening voltage-gated calcium channels. (3) Released calcium ions (Ca^{2+}) draw acetylcholine (ACh) vesicles to the neural membrane, (4) where they fuse with the membrane and empty a quantum of ACh into the synaptic space. The ACh binds to ACh receptors (AChR) on the postsynaptic muscle membrane. (5) The AChR responds by opening channels for the influx of sodium ions (Na^+), (6) with subsequent depolarization of the motor endplate. The resulting action potential leads to contraction of the muscle fiber.

or membrane attack complex (MAC). This results in lysis of the postsynaptic membrane, causing loss of the AChR (Figure 2.2).[5] In fact, elevated MAC levels have been demonstrated in the plasma of

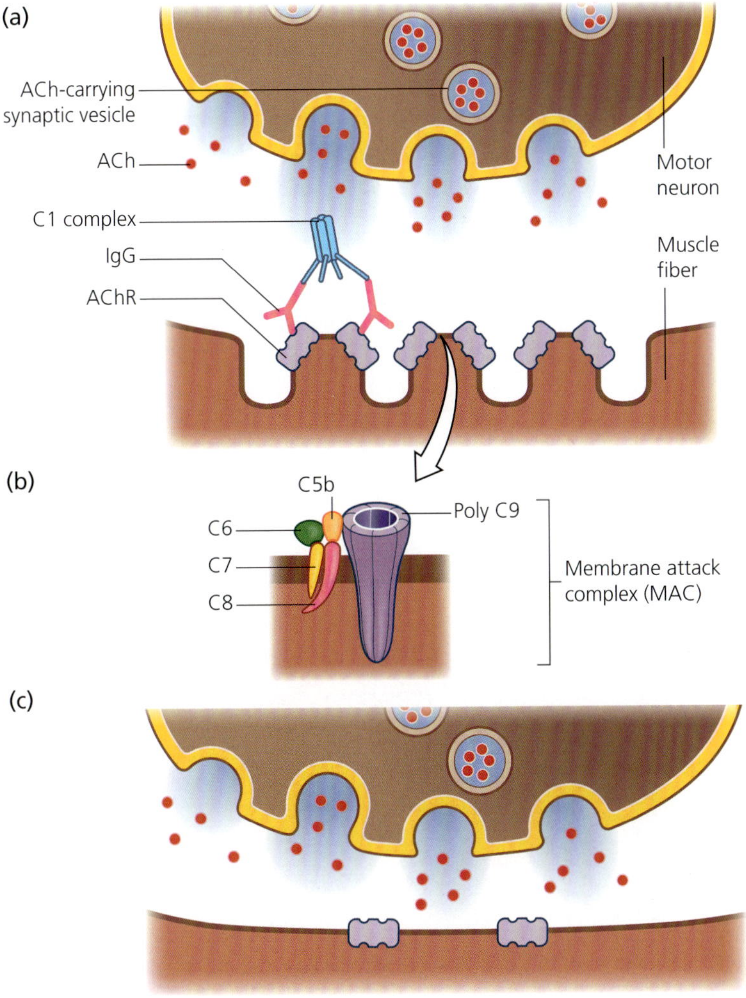

Figure 2.2 Binding and activation of complement. (a) The IgG antibody binds to the AChR, (b) activating the terminal complement sequence (C5b–9) and forming a membrane attack complex (MAC). (c) This triggers degeneration of the postsynaptic NMJ, which affects depolarization of the muscle membrane.

patients with MG.[6] 'Binding' antibodies are the most common type found in patients with MG.

Accelerated internalization and degradation of acetylcholine receptors. A key mechanism of disease pathology in MG is the modulation, internalization and eventual destruction of AChRs at the NMJ by the crosslinking of AChR-specific autoantibodies (Figure 2.3). This process is known as antigenic modulation.[4]

Direct blockade of acetylcholine receptors by antibodies. 'Blocking' antibodies are the second most common type found in patients with MG. These antibodies block the binding of ACh to AChRs on the muscle endplate (Figure 2.4).

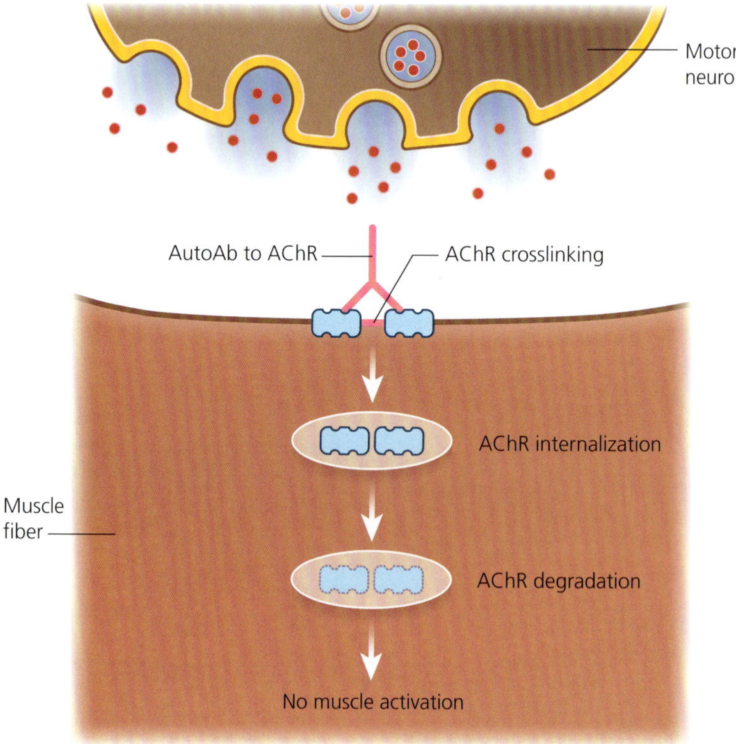

Figure 2.3 Antigenic modulation. Cross-linking of two acetylcholine receptor (AChR)-modulating autoantibodies leads to accelerated endocytosis and degradation of AChR, which reduces AChRs at the neuromuscular junction and reduces muscle activation. AutoAb, autoantibody.

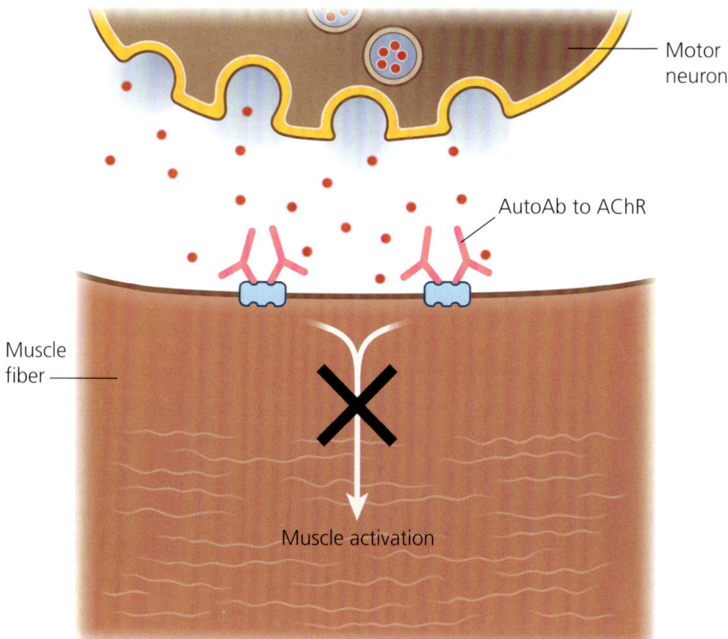

Figure 2.4 Functional blockade of acetylcholine receptors by antibodies. Antibodies bind to AChR binding sites, thus preventing binding of ACh with the receptor, causing failure of neuromuscular transmission. AutoAb, autoantibody.

Impaired neuromuscular transmission. As a result of the pathological processes described above, the postsynaptic membrane becomes simplified, with a reduction in the number of AChRs and junctional folds and a reduced safety factor in neuromuscular transmission, ultimately leading to impaired neuromuscular transmission.[7]

Muscle-specific receptor tyrosine kinase antibodies. Although most patients with generalized MG have antibodies to AChR (see below), a minority of patients without AChR antibodies have antibodies to the muscle-specific receptor tyrosine kinase (MuSK). As discussed in Chapter 1, a higher percentage of patients with treatment-refractory MG have been found to have MuSK antibodies than those who respond to treatment. The disease can be particularly severe in patients with MuSK antibodies (see below).

At present it is unclear how MuSK antibodies cause MG, but it is possible that MuSK antibodies alter AChR density or number. MuSK signaling is crucial for the development, long-term maintenance and stabilization of the postsynaptic portion of the NMJ. The antibodies in MuSK MG are largely of the IgG4 subclass and have been demonstrated in vitro to block the assembly and activation of MuSK. In animal models, administration of MuSK antibodies has resulted in reduced postsynaptic AChRs, disturbed synaptic alignment, reduced synaptic potentials and impaired muscle activation.[8]

Role of the thymus. Approximately 75% of patients who undergo thymectomy are found to have thymic pathology. Of these, 15% are discovered to have thymoma, and the remainder have evidence of lymphoid hyperplasia.[9] Myoid cells are located in the thymus gland, and thymus tissue from patients with MG has been found to be enriched with AChR-reactive T cells.[10] The close interaction between lymphocytes and myoid cells in the thymus, together with a yet-to-be-discovered stimulus that disrupts normal immune tolerance, may lead to the autoimmune response triggering MG.

Classification

MG can be classified in a variety of ways:

- by disease type
- by antibody status
- by disease severity.

Classification by disease type. Ocular MG, which causes only ptosis and/or diplopia, occurs in approximately 15% of cases; generalized disease occurs in the remainder.[11]

Classification by antibody status

Antibodies to AChR. As noted above, MG is most often caused by antibodies to the AChR. This is the case for 85% of cases of generalized disease and approximately 50% of cases of purely ocular MG. Antibodies to AChR may be of the binding, blocking or modulating type, with binding being the most common. AChR antibodies are highly specific for the diagnosis of MG, although the degree of elevation in titers has never been found to correlate with the severity of disease.[12] Antibody titers may decline with immunosuppressive treatment within an individual, although the reliability of determining treatment effect is less robust.

Antibodies to muscle receptor tyrosine kinase (MuSK) occur in about 7% of cases of generalized MG but are rarely reported in isolated ocular disease.[13] MuSK-antibody-positive MG is a distinct clinical subset of the disease, almost always seen in adults, more frequently in women, and never in conjunction with thymic disease.[13] There is predominant involvement of the bulbar muscles, often with concurrent neck and respiratory muscle weakness.[14] Ocular and limb muscle weakness is less common than in AChR-antibody-related disease but is certainly seen in this population. Most patients can actually worsen on treatment with acetylcholinesterase inhibitors such as pyridostigmine.

In general, treatment-refractory MG and myasthenic crises are more common in this subset of the disease.

Seronegative for AChR or MuSK antibodies. When AChR or MuSK antibodies are not detected, patients are diagnosed with MG by clinical or electrodiagnostic means (typically with repetitive nerve stimulation or single fiber electromyography; see page 25–26) and are classified as 'double seronegative' or 'seronegative'. Included in this group are a small percentage of patients with antibodies only to 'clustered' AChRs. These antibodies can only be detected using cell-based assays, which, in contrast to standard diagnostic antibody tests, allow for the detection of antibodies that bind to AChRs that are clustered in a natural membrane environment, as they are at the NMJ. These patients are more likely to be younger and have milder disease than other patients with MG.[15]

Other antibodies. Antibodies to lipoprotein-related protein 4 (LRP4), agrin and cortactin have recently been found in a small percentage of patients with MG.[16–18] Further discovery of pathogenic antibodies and improvements in antibody detection are likely to decrease the percentage of patients who are ultimately diagnosed with seronegative MG.

Classification by disease severity. Osserman was the first to classify patients with MG according to disease severity.[19] The most commonly used modification of the original classification scheme is as follows:

- Group I – ocular
- Group IIA – mild generalized
- Group IIB – moderate-to-severe generalized
- Group III – acute, severe, developing over weeks to months
- Group IV – late, severe, with marked bulbar involvement.

This classification has several notable limitations, including the indistinct descriptive wording and lack of clear distinctions between groups. This classification system also fails to include a category for patients in clinical remission or those in crisis.

A task force of the Myasthenia Gravis Foundation of America (MGFA) subsequently developed a refined classification system (Table 2.1) that is more clinically descriptive and provides a clearer distinction between groups.[20,21]

TABLE 2.1

MGFA clinical classification of myasthenia gravis

Class I	Any ocular muscle weakness; may have weakness of eye closure. All other muscle strength is normal
Class II	Mild weakness affecting muscles other than ocular muscles* Further classified as class IIa[a] and IIb[b]
Class III	Moderate weakness affecting muscles other than ocular muscles* Further classified as class IIIa[a] and IIIb[b]
Class IV	Severe weakness affecting muscles other than ocular muscles* Further classified as class IVa[a] and IVb[b]
Class V	Defined as intubation, with or without mechanical ventilation, except when employed during routine postoperative management. The use of a feeding tube without intubation places the patient in class IVb.

*May also have ocular muscle weakness of any severity.
[a]Predominantly affecting limb, axial muscles, or both. May also have lesser involvement of oropharyngeal muscles.
[b]Predominantly affecting oropharyngeal, respiratory muscles, or both. May also have lesser or equal involvement of limb, axial muscles, or both.
MGFA, Myasthenia Gravis Foundation of America.

Key points – pathophysiology and classification

- In myasthenia gravis (MG), pathogenic antibodies against acetylcholine receptors (AChRs) or muscle-specific receptor tyrosine kinase (MuSK) are responsible for the abnormal neuromuscular junction transmission leading to muscle weakness.
- Antibodies to AChRs reduce the number of AChRs by several pathological mechanisms including complement-activated damage, antigenic modulation leading to accelerated endocytosis and degradation of the AChR, and direct blockade of the receptor.
- Abnormal thymic pathology is associated with AChR-antibody-positive MG, particularly late-onset disease.
- About 7% of cases of generalized MG have antibodies to MuSK. This is a distinct clinical subset of the disease, which is generally more severe than AChR-antibody-positive MG, not associated with thymic pathology and more likely to be refractory to treatment.

References

1. Simpson J. Myasthenia gravis: a new hypothesis. *Scott Med J* 1960;5:419–36.

2. Lindstrom JM, Seybold ME, Lennon VA et al. Antibody to acetylcholine receptor in myasthenia gravis – prevalence, clinical correlates, and diagnostic value. *Neurology* 1976;26:1054–9.

3. Meriggioli MN, Sanders DB. Autoimmune myasthenia gravis: emerging clinical and biological heterogeneity. *Lancet Neurol* 2009;8:475–90.

4. Drachman DB, Adams RN, Stanley EF, Pestronk A. Mechanisms of acetylcholine receptor loss in myasthenia gravis. *J Neurol Neurosurg Psychiatry* 1980;43:601–10.

5. Engel AG, Arahata K. The membrane attack complex of complement at the endplate in myasthenia gravis. *Ann N Y Acad Sci* 1987;505:326–32.

6. Barohn RJ, Brey RL. Soluble terminal complement components in human myasthenia gravis. *Clin Neurol Neurosurg* 1993;95:285–90.

7. Engel AG, Tsujihata M, Lindstrom JM et al. The motor end plate in myasthenia gravis and in experimental autoimmune myasthenia gravis. A quantitative ultrastructural study. *Ann N Y Acad Sci* 1976;274:60–79.

8. Reddel SW, Morsch M, Phillips WD. Clinical and scientific aspects of muscle-specific tyrosine kinase-related myasthenia gravis. *Curr Opin Neurol* 2014;27:558–65.

9. Shelly S, Agmon-Levin N, Altman A, Shoenfeld Y. Thymoma and autoimmunity. *Cell Mol Immunol* 2011;8:199–202.

10. Kao I, Drachman DB. Thymic muscle cells bear acetylcholine receptors: possible relation to myasthenia gravis. *Science* 1977;195:74–5.

11. Grob D, Brunner N, Namba T, Pagala M. Lifetime course of myasthenia gravis. *Muscle Nerve* 2008;37:141–9.

12. Sanders DB, Burns TM, Cutter GR et al. Does change in acetylcholine receptor antibody level correlate with clinical change in myasthenia gravis? *Muscle Nerve* 2014;49:483–6.

13. Sanders DB, El-Salem K, Massey JM et al. Clinical aspects of MuSK antibody positive seronegative MG. *Neurology* 2003;60:1978–80.

14. Pasnoor M, Wolfe GI, Nations S et al. Clinical findings in MuSK-antibody positive myasthenia gravis: a U.S. experience. *Muscle Nerve* 2010;41:370–4.

15. Rodriguez Cruz PM, Al-Hajjar M, Huda S et al. Clinical features and diagnostic usefulness of antibodies to clustered acetylcholine receptors in the diagnosis of seronegative myasthenia gravis. *JAMA Neurol* 2015;72:642–9.

16. Gallardo E, Martinez-Hernàndez E, Titulaer MJ et al. Cortactin autoantibodies in myasthenia gravis. *Autoimmun Rev* 2014;13:1003–7.

17. Gasperi C, Melms A, Schoser B et al. Anti-agrin autoantibodies in myasthenia gravis. *Neurology* 2014; 82:1976–83.

18. Zhang B, Tzartos JS, Belimezi M et al. Autoantibodies to lipoprotein-related protein 4 in patients with double-negative myasthenia gravis. *Arch Neurol* 2012;69:445–51.

19. Osserman KE, Kornfeld P, Cohen E et al. Studies in myasthenia gravis; review of two hundred and eighty-two cases at the Mount Sinai Hopsital, New York City. *AMA Arch Intern Med* 1958;102:72–81.

20. Jaretzki A III, Barohn RJ, Ernstoff RM et al. Myasthenia gravis: recommendations for clinical research standards. *Ann Thorac Surg* 2000;70:327–34.

21. Barohn RJ. Standards of measurements in myasthenia gravis. *Ann N Y Acad Sci* 2003;998:432–9.

Further reading

Castleman B. The pathology of the thymus gland in myasthenia gravis. *Ann N Y Acad Sci* 1966;135:496–505.

3 Diagnosis and management: an overview

Clinical presentation

Myasthenia gravis (MG) is characterized by skeletal muscle weakness (Table 3.1). As with any disorder of neuromuscular transmission, the distinctive clinical feature of MG is the fluctuating nature of weakness that patients report – a phenomenon known as 'fatigability'. Symptoms of MG tend to worsen with concurrent illness, over-exertion of the muscle (e.g. fatigue from speaking or eating), the use of certain medications, and as the day progresses. The presentation of MG in any given patient is variable; not all patients will experience all of the symptoms described below.

Ocular symptoms. Approximately two-thirds of patients initially present with ocular symptoms.[1,2] Neurological examination often discloses evidence of ptosis or dysconjugate gaze on testing of

TABLE 3.1

Manifestations of myasthenia gravis by muscle type

Muscle	Principal manifestations
Ocular	Ptosis, diplopia
Bulbar	Dysarthria, dysphagia, dysphonia, tongue weakness, jaw weakness with impaired chewing
Facial	Difficulty with eye closure, conjunctival irritation, impaired smile
Neck	Difficulty holding head up
Respiratory	Orthopnea or dyspnea
Limb	Proximal limb and axial muscles tend to be weaker than distal extremity muscles; a minority of patients may experience predominantly distal upper extremity weakness

extraocular movements, which may demonstrate fatigability with sustained upward or lateral gaze. Weakness of the eye muscles is often asymmetric and variable – a combination of alternating ptosis and diplopia in any direction.

Generalized symptoms. The disease spreads beyond the eye muscle in over 80% of patients,[3] with a predilection for bulbar, facial, neck and proximal limb muscle involvement. Dysarthria or dysphonia may manifest after the patient speaks for a prolonged period of time. Testing of neck and limb muscles should likewise be done after a period of exercise to evaluate for evidence of fatigability. Respiratory muscles may also be affected, leading to dyspnea on exertion or orthopnea.

Myasthenic crisis. Roughly 15% of patients with MG will experience myasthenic crisis, defined as respiratory failure due to MG, most likely within the the first 2 years following symptom onset.[4] This necessitates intubation and mechanical ventilation until clinical improvement in strength occurs.

Diagnostic work-up

In most instances, the clinician can be confident about the diagnosis of MG based on a characteristic history and physical examination. However, one or more tests are routinely performed to confirm the clinical diagnosis.

Antibody testing. Testing for acetylcholine receptor (AChR) antibodies is always performed in patients suspected of having MG. If these antibodies are present, no further diagnostic testing is usually required other than to evaluate for the presence of a thymoma with either CT or MRI of the thorax.

AChR-antibody-negative patients with predominant bulbar involvement are often tested for muscle-specific receptor tyrosine kinase (MuSK) antibodies.[5] Testing for antibodies to the P/Q type voltage-gated calcium channel is also often performed in cases of AChR antibody negativity to rule out Lambert Eaton myasthenic syndrome.

In children with myasthenic features but with AChR-, clustered AChR- and MuSK-antibody negativity, congenital (genetic) myasthenic syndromes should be considered.

Electrophysiological tests. In cases of antibody negativity, a decrementing response on slow (3 Hz) repetitive nerve stimulation (Figure 3.1) or elevated jitter values on single fiber electromyography (Figure 3.2) may be necessary to confirm the diagnosis of MG.

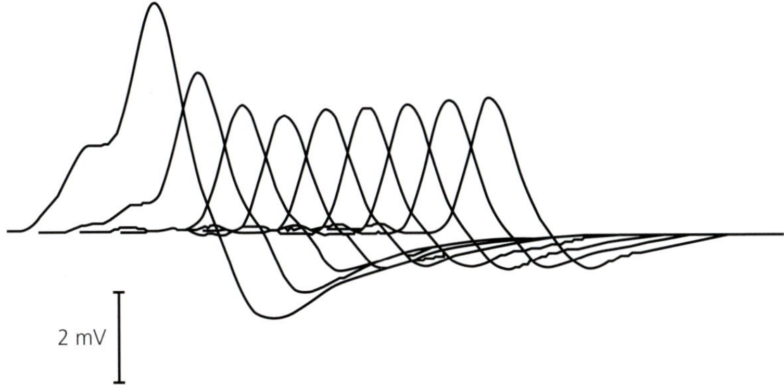

Figure 3.1 A typical smoothly decrementing response on a stable baseline to repetitive nerve stimulation in a patient with myasthenia gravis. The initial response is normal and the decrement is maximal in the fourth response. The responses then slowly increase.

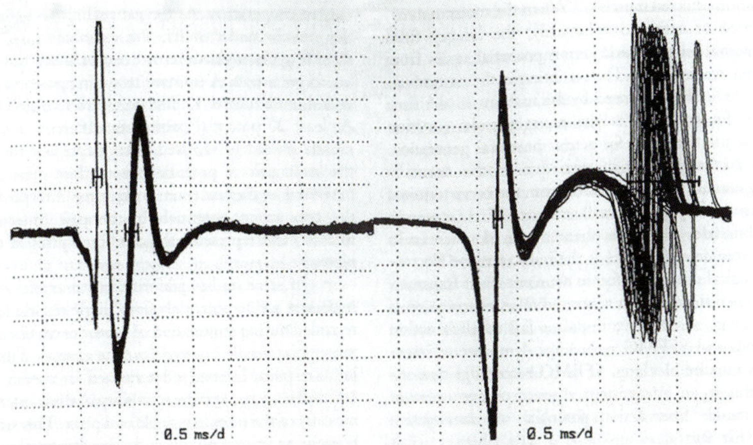

Figure 3.2 Single fiber electromyography. Two action potentials recorded from a patient with myasthenia gravis during voluntary activation of the muscle. Consecutive discharges are superimposed. Increased jitter is seen in the second potential.

It is worth noting that, while increased jitter on single fiber electromyography is very sensitive in patients with MG, it is not specific for the disease, therefore other causes of weakness should be ruled out. In addition, a decremental response on repetitive nerve stimuation may disappear in patients with MG in a muscle that is no longer clinically weak. In other words, lack of decrement in a muscle that is reported to be weak may indicate a cause other than MG.

Edrophonium test. A positive edrophonium test ('Tensilon test') can also be used to confirm the diagnosis. Patients with MG should show an improvement in muscular strength following administration of edrophonium, a very short-acting anticholinesterase, which therefore increases the effective amount of acetylcholine at the neuromuscular junction (NMJ).

Conventional management

The treatment of MG should be individualized according to the patient's disease severity and its effect on daily living and quality of life, comorbid medical conditions and personal preferences.

Acetylcholinesterase inhibitors have been used in the treatment of MG since 1934 when Walker successfully treated a patient with physostigmine for generalized disease.[6] These agents are often the initial therapeutic intervention in MG. They work by inhibiting the enzymatic hydrolysis of acetylcholine (ACh) at the synapse, allowing the neurotransmitter to accumulate at the NMJ, prolonging its activity and increasing the number of neurotransmitter and AChR interactions.

Pyridostigmine bromide is the preferred acetylcholinesterase inhibitor as it has a longer half-life and a more favorable side-effect profile than other available agents. Unfortunately, most patients with MG cannot be controlled on anticholinesterase medications alone and require treatment with either thymectomy or immunosuppressive or immunomodulatory therapy (Figure 3.3).

Corticosteroids were the first immunosuppressant drugs to be widely used in the treatment of MG. They produce significant clinical improvement in the vast majority of patients.[7] The response to

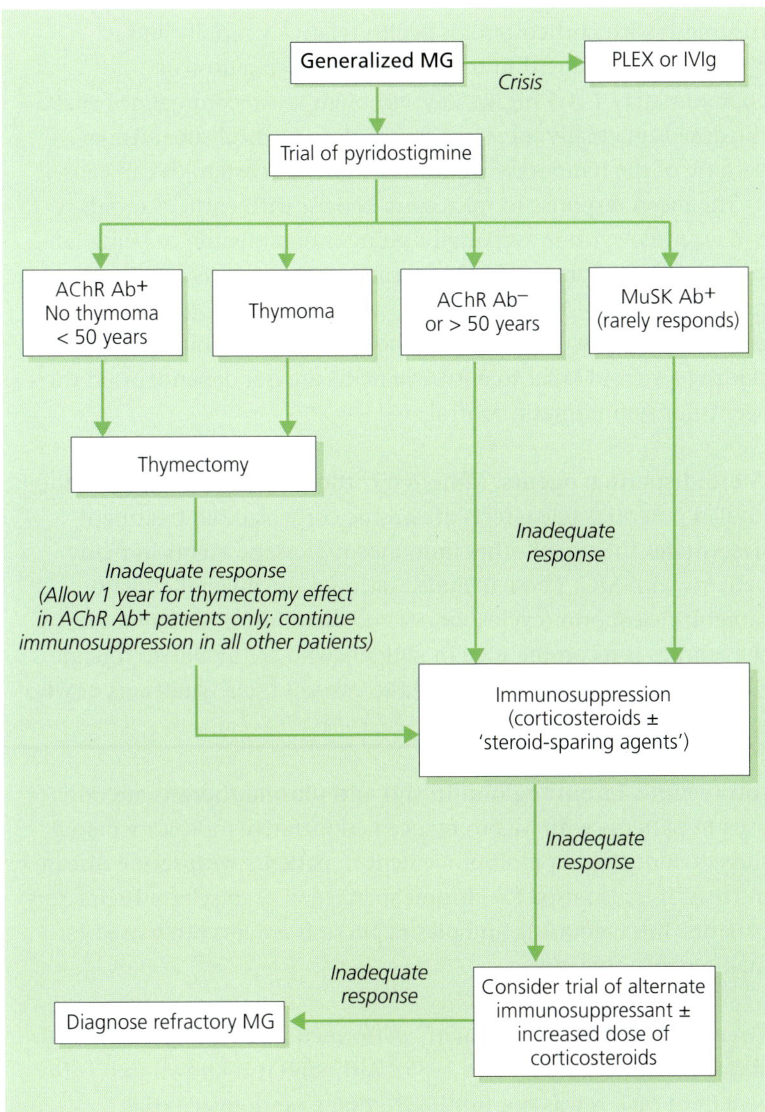

Figure 3.3 The treatment of generalized myasthenia gravis using conventional therapies, beginning with a trial of pyridostigmine bromide. Inadequate response to all conventional therapies leads to a diagnosis of refractory myasthenia gravis (MG). AChR Ab, acetylcholine receptor antibody; IVIg, intravenous immunoglobulin; MuSK Ab, muscle receptor tyrosine kinase antibody; PLEX, plasma exchange.

treatment with corticosteroids begins relatively rapidly and is typically observed within the first 2–4 weeks at a dose of approximately 1–1.5 mg/kg/day, although it is recommended that the dose is gradually increased under close medical supervision because of the temporary worsening that corticosteroids can cause.[7]

The mean response to maximum benefit with corticosteroids is 5–6 months,[7] with most patients going into remission or being left with only mild symptoms. Once reached, this dose is usually maintained for 1–3 months, with a slow taper thereafter. Some clinicians will discontinue acetylcholinesterase inhibitors before starting a steroid taper to ensure patients are not dependent on these agents for symptomatic control.

'Steroid-sparing' agents. Although corticosteroids are effective, the myriad potential side effects of chronic corticosteroid treatment necessitates the use of other immunosuppressant agents in many patients with MG. These include azathioprine, mycophenolate mofetil, ciclosporin (cyclosporine) and tacrolimus.[7] A trial of one of these drugs is recommended in patients who are unable to tolerate the dose of corticosteroid required to control their symptoms or who relapse during a steroid taper.

Intravenous immunoglobulin (Ig) and plasmapheresis are often used in patients with MG to reduce perioperative morbidity before surgery, inducing rapid improvement in patients with severe disease or in crisis. It is also used for chronic management in selected refractory patients. Intravenous Ig and plasmapheresis are less often used for maintenance therapy.

Thymectomy has been regularly performed for MG in patients with and without thymoma since 1939.[8] Although it is known to be of benefit in MG, it was not until 2016 that a randomized trial demonstrated clear benefit of thymectomy in non-thymomatous MG.[9] Thymectomy is of greatest benefit in patients younger than 40 years of age, but maximal benefit may not be seen until 3 years after surgery.

Management of refractory patients

When patients with MG are deemed to be refractory to conventional treatment (see page 8), consideration of additional therapeutic options is warranted in order to improve quality of life, reduce morbidity and prevent life-threatening crises and death. While there are no evidence-based guidelines, recently published international consensus guidelines for the management of MG recommend referral to a physician or center with expertise in the management of the disorder, and that treatment with chronic intravenous immunoglobulin or plasma exchange, cyclophosphamide or rituximab should be considered.[10] Other treatment options are emerging.[11]

Key points – diagnosis and management: an overview

- Myasthenia gravis (MG) is characterized by skeletal muscle weakness and fatigability. It can affect the ocular, bulbar, facial, neck, respiratory and limb muscles.
- The symptoms of MG may be exacerbated by concurrent illness, over-exertion of the muscle, the use of certain medications, and as the day progresses.
- All patients suspected of having MG should be tested for acetylcholine receptor (AChR) antibodies. If these antibodies are present, no further diagnostic testing is usually required other than the use of imaging to determine if a thymoma is present.
- AChR-antibody-negative patients with predominant bulbar involvement are often tested for muscle-specific receptor tyrosine kinase (MuSK) antibodies and, where available, antibodies to clustered AChR. (It should be noted, however, that clustered AChR antibody testing is available only at a few specialist centers, and is not routinely performed in general laboratories.)
- Patients who are antibody negative should be tested for a decrementing response on repetitive nerve stimulation, elevated jitter values on single fiber electromyography or a positive edrophonium test.
- Acetylcholinesterase inhibitors are often the initial therapeutic intervention in patients with MG.
- Most patients with MG require additional treatment with either thymectomy or immunosuppressive or immunomodulatory therapy.
- Consideration of additional therapeutic options is warranted for patients who are identified as being refractory to conventional treatment.

References

1. Oosterhuis HJ. The ocular signs and symptoms of myasthenia gravis. *Doc Ophthalmol* 1982;52:363–78.

2. Conti-Fine BM, Milani M, Kaminski HJ. Myasthenia gravis: past, present, and future. *J Clin Invest* 2006;116:2843–54.

3. Grob D, Brunner N, Namba T, Pagala M. Lifetime course of myasthenia gravis. *Muscle Nerve* 2008;37:141–9.

4. Ahmed S, Kirmani JF, Janjua N et al. An update on myasthenic crisis. *Curr Treat Options Neurol* 2005;7:129–41.

5. Evoli A, Tonali PA, Padua L et al. Clinical correlates with anti-MuSK antibodies in generalized seronegative myasthenia gravis. *Brain* 2003;126:2304–11.

6. Walker MB. Treatment of myasthenia with physostigmine. *Lancet* 1934;1:1200–1.

7. Silvestri NJ, Wolfe GI. Myasthenia gravis. *Semin Neurol* 2012;32:215–26.

8. Blalock A, Mason MF, Morgan HJ, Riven SS. Myasthenia gravis and tumors of the thymic region: report of a case in which the tumor was removed. *Ann Surgery* 1939;110:544–61.

9. Wolfe GI, Kaminski HJ, Aban IB et al. Randomized trial of thymectomy in myasthenia gravis. *N Engl J Med* 2016;375:511–22.

10 Sanders DB, Wolfe GI, Benatar M et al. International consensus guidance for management of myasthenia gravis. Executive summary. *Neurology* 2016;87:419–25.

11. Silvestri NJ. Wolfe GI. Treatment-refractory myasthenia gravis. *J Clin Neuromuscul Dis* 2014;15:167–78.

Further reading

Bershad EM, Feen ES, Suarez JI. Myasthenia gravis crisis. *South Med J* 2008;101:63–9.

Johns TR. Long-term cortocosteroid treatment of myasthenia gravis. *Ann N Y Acad Sci* 1987;505:568–83.

Philips LH 2nd. The epidemiology of myasthenia gravis. *Ann N Y Acad Sci* 2003;998:407–12.

Sussman J, Farrugia ME, Maddison P et al. Myasthenia gravis: Association of British Neurologists' management guidelines. *Pract Neurol* 2015;15:199–206.

4 Assessment of disease severity and treatment response

Although myasthenia gravis (MG) is a very treatable disease in most patients, approximately 10–15% have very difficult-to-control disease. These patients often experience disabling symptoms that lead to poor quality of life and are prone to life-threatening crises.

Given the fluctuations in severity of symptoms in patients with MG, there are inherent difficulties in assessing baseline disease severity and response to treatment. Electrophysiological studies, disease severity rating scales and patient-reported outcome measures are all tools with which disease activity and response to treatment have been measured in MG.

Measuring antibodies

Intuitively, the measurement of acetylcholine receptor (AChR) antibody titers serves as an attractive biomarker to discern disease activity and response to treatment in patients with MG. However, it is generally accepted that there is no reliable correlation between serum AChR antibody titers and clinical severity in generalized MG. A recent study using a commercial assay noted a high positive predictive value but a low negative predictive value when correlating titers with several validated outcome measures in MG. The measurement of AChR antibody levels is therefore likely to be of limited benefit when attempting to discern the level of disease activity.[1]

Research need. Better prognostic biomarkers for MG are needed to more sensitively determine which treatments might work better for specific patients, to better assess the response to treatment over time and for use in clinical trial design in studies of MG.

Electrophysiological tests

Measurement of jitter on single fiber electromyography (SFEMG) has shown promise as a useful biomarker of disease activity in MG (see page 25–26). One recent study found that jitter is a sensitive measure of disease severity in MG; absolute or percentage change in mean jitter from one electrophysiological study to another in a given patient has a potential role as a biomarker.[2] Another study showed that high jitter values on SFEMG and decrement values on repetitive nerve stimulation were associated with more severe disease, as determined by more frequent subjective and objective measures of muscle strength and worse quantitative MG score (see below).[3]

Clinical rating instruments

Several clinical rating instruments have been developed to measure disease severity and quality of life, in patients with MG.

The quantitative MG score (QMG) is the best studied objective outcome measure in MG, and it has been used in many drug trials in MG. It is a severity score, determined from measurement of 13 objective items (Table 4.1), with measures varying between 0 (normal) to 39 (maximum severity). The QMG can be completed in 20–30 minutes, and the only specialized equipment required is a spirometer and handheld dynamometer. Spirometry, dynamometry and quantitative timed tests can also be useful longitudinally in individual patients even when the total QMG does not change. The Myasthenia Gravis Foundation of America (MGFA) task force recommended that the QMG be used in all prospective studies of therapy for MG.[4]

The MG activities of daily living score (MG-ADL) is a simple eight-point questionnaire, designed to complement the QMG, which enquires about common symptoms reported by patients with MG (Table 4.2). Widely used in many studies, the MG-ADL correlates well with the QMG and can serve as a measure of efficacy in clinical trials.[5] No specialized training is required to administer the scale, which can be completed in less than 10 minutes.

The MG composite scale (MGC) consists of test items that measure symptoms and signs of MG, with weighted response options to highlight aspects of weakness that may be more serious such as bulbar and respiratory function. It was devised using individual test items taken from existing MG-specific scales based on their performance during two clinical trials of mycophenolate mofetil for the treatment of MG.[6]

TABLE 4.1

Quantitative myasthenia gravis score

	None (0)	Mild (1)	Moderate (2)	Severe (3)
1. Double vision on lateral gaze, R or L (s)	61	11–60	1–10	Spontaneous
2. Ptosis on upward gaze (s)	61	11–60	1-10	Spontaneous
3. Facial muscles	Normal lid closure	Complete, weak, some resistance	Complete, without resistance	Incomplete
4. Swallowing 120 mL (4 oz) of water	Normal	Minimal coughing or throat clearing	Severe coughing/ choking*	Cannot swallow (test not attempted)
5. Speech after counting aloud from 1–50 (onset of dysarthria)	None at #50	Dysarthria at #30–49	Dysarthria at #10–29	Dysarthria at #9
6. Right arm stretched at 90° when sitting (s)	240	90–239	10–89	0–9
7. Left arm stretched at 90° when sitting (s)	240	90–239	10–89	0–9
8. Vital capacity,† best of 3 (% predicted)	≥ 80%	65–79%	50–64%	< 50%
9. Right hand grip (best of 2) (kgW)	≥ 45 M ≥ 30 F	15–44 10–29	5–14 5–9	0–4 0–4
10. Left hand grip (best of 2) (kgW)	≥ 35 M ≥ 25 F	15–34 10–24	5–14 5–9	0–4 0–4
11. Head, lifted at 45° when supine (s)	120	30–119	1–29	0
12. Right leg stretched at 45° when supine (s)	100	31–99	1–30	0
13. Left leg stretched at 45° when supine (s)	100	31–99	1–30	0

QMG total is out of 39. *Or nasal regurgitation. †Using mouthpiece or facemask. F, female; L, left; M, male; R, right; s, seconds. Adapted from Barohn RJ. *The Quantitative Myasthenia Gravis (QMG) Test: The Manual.* Myasthenia Gravis Foundation of America, 2000. myasthenia.org/LinkClick.aspx?fileticket=9U5kP6SfCJs%3D&tabid=125, last accessed 27 February 2018.

TABLE 4.2

Myasthenia gravis activities of daily living score

	0	1	2	3	Insert score (0, 1, 2 or 3)
1. Talking	Normal	Intermittent slurring or nasal speech	Constant slurring or nasal speech, but can be understood	Difficult to understand speech	
2. Chewing	Normal	Fatigue with solid food	Fatigue with soft food	Gastric tube	
3. Swallowing	Normal	Rare episode of choking	Frequent choking necessitating changes in diet	Gastric tube	
4. Breathing	Normal	Shortness of breath with exertion	Shortness of breath at rest	Ventilator dependence	
5. Impairment of ability to brush teeth or comb hair	None	Extra effort, but no rest periods needed	Rest periods needed	Cannot do one of these functions	
6. Impairment of ability to arise from a chair	None	Mild, sometimes uses arms	Moderate, always uses arms	Severe, requires assistance	
7. Double vision	None	Occurs, but not daily	Daily, but not constant	Constant	
8. Eyelid droop	None	Occurs, but not daily	Daily, but not constant	Constant	
				MG-ADL score total (items 1–8) /24	

The MGC consists of a combination of physician-measured signs and patient-reported symptoms (Table 4.3). It is easy to administer, usually taking less than 5 minutes to complete, and covers the ten important functional domains most frequently affected in MG, which have been appropriately weighted; it has been validated.[7]

The MG quality of life 15 scale (MG-QOL15). Measures of health-related quality of life attempt to ascertain a patient's subjective determination of the extent of dysfunction caused by disease and their degree of satisfaction or dissatisfaction with that dysfunction. MG-QOL15 is a 15-item MG-specific self-administered scale, the test items of which address MG-specific psychological well-being and social functioning. It is meant to inform the treating physician about a particular patient's perception of the extent of dysfunction specifically due to MG, and the degree of satisfaction or dissatisfaction with that dysfunction, which can then be used to help guide treatment decisions.[8] It can also be used to follow an individual patient's response over time to assist in assessing the degree of disease severity and to determine the efficacy of treatment, controlling for other potential confounding factors. In addition, like the other scales discussed, the MG-QOL15 has served to assist in following groups of patients with MG over time in clinical trials.

The scale has been revised using Rasch analysis (MG-QOL15R), which has slightly improved clinimetric properties and improved face and content validity (Table 4.4).[9] Both scales are validated; however, the MG-QOL15R is preferred given the better content validity and because it is somewhat easier to interpret in the clinical setting. Both scales take less than 5 minutes to administer.

The MG impairment index (MGII) was recently developed, importantly taking into account patient input in construction of the scale.[10] Using this patient-centered approach, the scale aims to measure the impairments that are judged to be most relevant by patients, particularly those that may be triggered by activity or that fluctuate and might not be easily assessed during a clinic visit. Like the MGC, however, several objective examination items were also incorporated into this scale. The MGII was found to have excellent reliability and is easy to implement. MGII scores have been found to

TABLE 4.3

Myasthenia gravis composite score

Ptosis, upward gaze – physician exam (s)	> 45 **(0)**	11–45 **(1)**	1–10 **(2)**	Immediate **(3)**
Double vision on lateral gaze, L or R – physician exam (s)	> 45 **(0)**	11–45 **(1)**	1–10 **(3)**	Immediate **(4)**
Eye closure – physician exam	Normal **(0)**	Mild weakness; can be forced open with effort **(0)**	Moderate weakness; can be forced open easily **(1)**	Severe weakness; unable to keep eyes closed **(2)**
Talking – patient history	Normal **(0)**	Intermittent slurring or nasal speech **(2)**	Constant slurring or nasal speech, but can be understood **(4)**	Difficult to understand speech **(6)**
Chewing – patient history	Normal **(0)**	Fatigue with solid food **(2)**	Fatigue with soft food **(4)**	Gastric tube **(6)**
Swallowing – patient history	Normal **(0)**	Rare episode of choking or trouble swallowing **(2)**	Frequent trouble swallowing e.g. necessitating changes in diet **(5)**	Gastric tube **(6)**
Breathing (thought to be caused by MG)	Normal **(0)**	Shortness of breath with exertion **(2)**	Shortness of breath at rest **(4)**	Ventilator dependence **(9)**
Neck flexion or extension (weakest) –physician exam	Normal **(0)**	Mild weakness **(1)**	Moderate weakness (~50% weak, ± 15%) **(3)**	Severe weakness **(4)**
Shoulder abduction – physician exam	Normal **(0)**	Mild weakness **(2)**	Moderate weakness (~50% weak, ± 15%) **(4)**	Severe weakness **(5)**
Hip flexion – physician exam	Normal **(0)**	Mild weakness **(2)**	Moderate weakness (~50% weak, ± 15%) **(4)**	Severe weakness **(5)**

L, left; R, right; s, seconds.

TABLE 4.4

Myasthenia gravis quality of life 15R (MGQOL15R) score

Please indicate how true each statement has been (over the past few weeks)	Not at all 0	Some-what 1	Very much 2
1. I am frustrated by my MG			
2. I have trouble with my eyes because of my MG (e.g. double vision)			
3. I have trouble eating because of MG			
4. I have limited my social activity because of my MG			
5. My MG limits my ability to enjoy hobbies and fun activities			
6. I have trouble meeting the needs of my family because of my MG			
7. I have to make plans around my MG			
8. I am bothered by limitations in performing my work (include work at home) because of my MG			
9. I have difficulty speaking due to MG			
10. I have lost some personal independence because of my MG (e.g. driving, shopping, running errands)			
11. I am depressed about my MG			
12. I have trouble walking due to MG			
13. I have trouble getting around public places because of my MG			
14. I feel overwhelmed by my MG			
15. I have trouble performing my personal grooming needs due to MG			

Total MGQOL15R score =

correlate well with other validated scales discussed above, including the QMG, MG-ADL, MGC and MG-QOL15.

The MGFA assessment of post-intervention status (PIS) designates the clinical state of patients with MG at any time point after initiation of a particular treatment and can be used for routine follow-up in the clinic or in formal clinical trials (Table 4.5).

TABLE 4.5

MGFA post-intervention status

Complete stable remission (CSR)

- No symptoms or signs of myasthenia gravis (MG) for at least 1 year and no therapy for MG during that time
- No weakness of any muscle on careful examination by someone skilled in the evaluation of neuromuscular disease. Isolated weakness of eyelid closure is accepted

Pharmacological remission (PR)

- The same criteria as for CSR except continuation of some form of therapy for MG
- Patients taking cholinesterase inhibitors are excluded because use of these agents suggests the presence of weakness

Minimal manifestations (MM)

- No symptoms of functional limitations from MG but some weakness on examination of some muscles
- This class recognizes that some patients who otherwise meet the definition of CSR or PR have weakness that is only detectable by careful examination
  - MM-0 No MG treatment for at least 1 year
  - MM-1 Continuing some form of immunosuppression but no cholinesterase inhibitors or other symptomatic therapy
  - MM-2 Only low-dose cholinesterase inhibitors (< 120 mg pyridostigmine/day) for at least 1 year
  - MM-3 Cholinesterase inhibitors or other symptomatic therapy and some form of immunosuppression during the past year

(CONTINUED)

TABLE 4.5 (CONTINUED)

MGFA post-intervention status

Change in status

Improved (I) A substantial decrease in pretreatment clinical manifestations or a sustained substantial reduction in MG medications as defined in the protocol. In prospective studies, this should be defined as a specific decrease in the quantitative MG score (QMG)

Unchanged (U) No substantial change in pretreatment clinical manifestations or reduction in MG medications as defined in the protocol. In prospective studies, this should be defined in terms of a maximum change in the QMG

Worse (W) A substantial increase in pretreatment clinical manifestations or a substantial increase in MG medications as defined in the protocol. In prospective studies, this should be defined as a specific increase in the QMG

Exacerbation (E) Patients who have fulfilled criteria of CSR, PR, or MM but subsequently developed clinical findings greater than permitted by these criteria

Died of MG (D of MG) Patients who died of MG, of complications of MG therapy, or within 30 days of thymectomy. List the cause

MGFA, Myasthenia Gravis Foundation of America.

The PIS should be determined by a clinician skilled in the evaluation of patients with MG since it is based on careful clinical evaluation, taking into account patient-reported symptoms and signs.

Monitoring treatment response

The frequency of monitoring will depend on the patient's response to therapy and fluctuations in disease activity. Unstable patients may be assessed every 1–2 months depending on the severity of their symptoms and admitted to hospital if more aggressive treatment, such as plasma exchange or intravenous immunoglobulin, is required.

Before patients with MG are deemed to be refractory to treatment, it is also important to rule out other factors that may be exacerbating the disease, such as non-adherence to medication, infection or, commonly, non-myasthenic causes of fatigue (Figure 4.1).

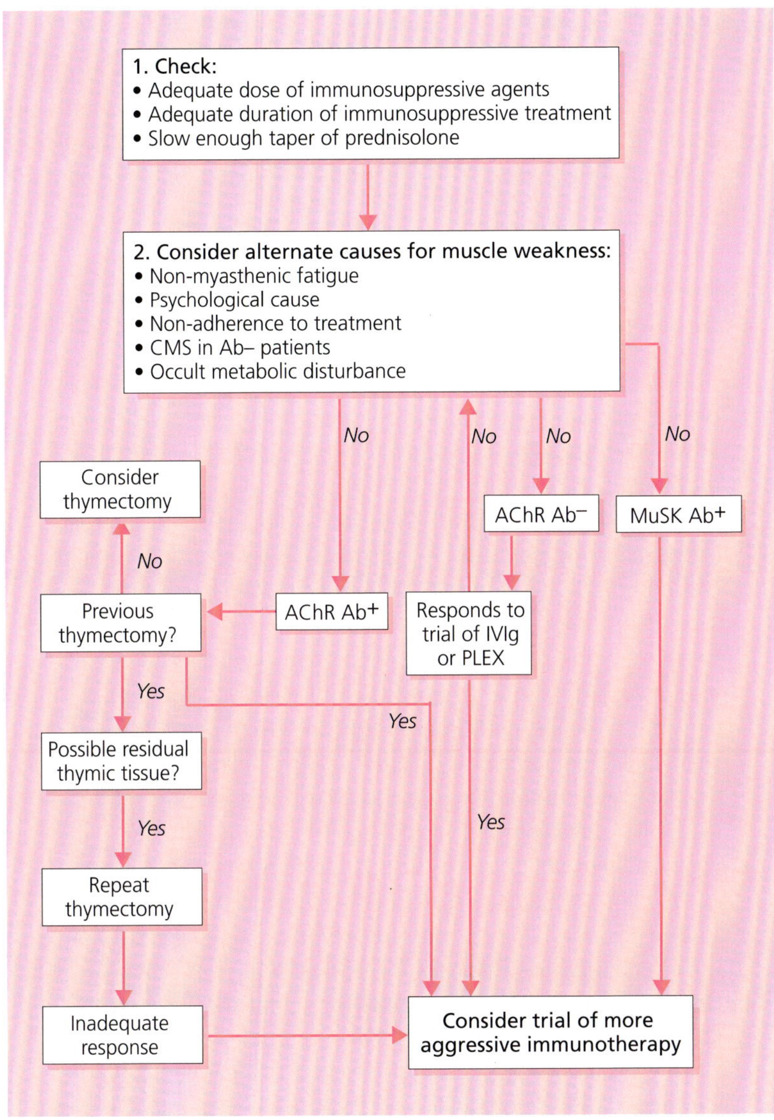

Figure 4.1 The management of patients who do not respond to conventional treatment. AChR Ab, acetylcholine receptor antibody; CMS, congenital myasthenia syndrome; IVIg, intravenous immunoglobulin; MuSK Ab, muscle receptor tyrosine kinase antibody; PLEX, plasma exchange; +, positive; –, negative.

The future

When patients with MG are deemed to be refractory to conventional treatment, aggressive treatments may be needed to improve quality of life, reduce morbidity and prevent life-threatening crises and death. Development of new treatments should be evaluated for these patients in the future.

Key points – assessment of disease severity and treatment response

- Electrophysiological studies, disease severity rating scales and patient-reported outcome measures are all tools with which disease activity and response to treatment can be measured in myasthenia gravis (MG).
- There is no reliable correlation between serum acetylcholine receptor (AChR) antibody titers and clinical severity in generalized MG; better prognostic biomarkers for MG are needed to better assess response to treatment over time.
- Measurement of jitter on single fiber electromyography (SFEMG) may be a useful biomarker of disease activity in MG. Absolute or percentage change in mean jitter from one electrophysiological study to another has a potential role as a biomarker provided the parameters of the study, such as time of day and time after medication, are kept the same.
- The quantitative MG score, which can be completed in 20–30 minutes and requires no specialized equipment, is the best studied objective outcome measure in MG. It is recommended for use in all prospective studies of therapy for MG.
- Other useful tools for assessing response to treatment include the MG activities of daily living score (MG-ADL), MG composite scale (MGC), revised MG quality of life 15 scale (MG-QOL15R), MG impairment index (MGII) and MGFA assessment of post-intervention status (PIS).

References

1. Sanders DB, Burns TM, Cutter GR et al. Does change in acetylcholine receptor antibody level correlate with clinical change in myasthenia gravis? *Muscle Nerve* 2014;49:483–6.

2. Sanders DB, Massey JM. Does change in neuromuscular jitter predict or correlate with clinical change in MG? *Muscle Nerve* 2017;56:45–50.

3. Abraham A, Breiner A, Barnett C et al. Electrophysiological testing is correlated with myasthenia gravis severity. *Muscle Nerve* 2017 doi:10.1002/mus.25539 [Epub ahead of print]

4. Jaretzki A III, Barohn RJ, Ernstoff RM et al. Myasthenia gravis: recommendations for clinical research standards. *Ann Thoracic Surg* 2000;70:327–34.

5. Wolfe GI, Herbelin L, Nations SP et al. Myasthenia gravis activities of daily living profile. *Neurology* 1999;52:1487–9.

6. Burns TM, Conaway MR, Cutter GR et al. Construction of an efficient evaluative instrument for myasthenia gravis: the MG Composite. *Muscle Nerve* 2008;38:1553–62.

7. Burns TM, Conaway MR, Sanders DB. The MG Composite: a valid and reliable outcome measure for myasthenia gravis. *Neurology* 2010;74:1434–40.

8. Burns TM, Grouse CK, Wolfe GI et al. The MG-QOL15 for following the health-related quality of life in patients with myasthenia gravis. *Muscle Nerve* 2011;43:14–18.

9. Burns TM, Sadjadi R, Utsugisawa K et al. International clinimetric evaluation of the MG-QOL15, resulting in slight revision and subsequent validation of the MG-QOL15r. *Muscle Nerve* 2016;54:1015–22.

10. Barnett C, Bril V, Kapral M et al. Development and validation of the Myasthenia Gravis Impairment Index. *Neurology* 2016;87:879–86.

Useful resources

European Association of Myasthenia Gravis Patients' Associations
www.eumga.eu

Myasthenia Alliance Australia
www.myastheniaallianceaustralia.com.au

The Australian Myasthenic Association in NSW Inc.
Tel: (02) 4283 2815
www.myasthenia.org.au

Myasthenia Gravis Association of Queensland Inc.
Toll-free: 1 800 802 568
www.mgaq.org.au

Myasthenia Gravis Foundation of America
Tel: 1 800 541 5454
www.myasthenia.org

Myasthenia Gravis Society of Canada
Tel: +1 905 642 2545
www.mgcanada.org

Myaware UK
Tel: +44 (0)1332 290219
info@myaware.org
www.myaware.org

National Organization for Rare Disorders (USA)
Tel: +1 203 744 0100
Patient services: 1 800 999 6673
https://rarediseases.org/rare-diseases/myastenia-gravis/

Rare Disease UK
www.raredisease.org.uk

Index

acetylcholine receptor
antibodies 13–17, 18–19, 24
to clustered AChR 19
and response to treatment 32
acetylcholine receptors (AChR) 13
acetylcholinesterase inhibitors 19, 26
activities of daily living score 33, 35
age 8–10, 24
antibodies 21
to AChR 13–17, 18–19, 24, 32
to clustered AChR 19
to MuSK 10, 17–18, 19, 24
not found/other 19, 24
antigenic modulation 16
assessment 32–42
biomarkers 32–3
clinical rating instruments 33–40
post-intervention status 39–40
treatment-refractory MG 40–1

bulbar symptoms 19, 23

children with MG 10, 24
classification 18–20
clinical presentation 23–4
clinical rating instruments 33–40
complement 13–16
corticosteroids 10, 26–8

diabetes mellitus 10
diagnosis 23–8
presentation 23–4
tests 19, 24–6
diplopia 18, 23–4, 34, 35, 37
dysarthria 24, 34, 35, 37
dyslipidemia 10

early-onset MG 8, 24
edrophonium test 26
electrophysiological tests 25–6, 32–3, 42
epidemiology 7–10
ethnicity 10
fatigability 23, 24
females 8–10

gender 8–10
genetics 10, 24
geography 10

HLA antigens 10

immunotherapy 28, 29
incidence 7–8

juvenile MG 8, 24
males 8, 9
management 26–9, 40–1, 42
acetylcholinesterase inhibitors 19, 26
assessment of disease 32–41
corticosteroids 10, 26–8
IVIG/plasmapheresis 28
other immuno-suppressants 28
refractory disease 19, 29, 41, 42
thymectomy 28
treatment algorithms 27, 41
MG activities of daily living score 33, 35
MG composite scale 33, 36, 37
MG impairment index 36, 39
MG quality of life 15 scale 36, 38
muscle-specific receptor tyrosine kinase (MuSK) antibodies 10, 17–8, 19, 24

myasthenic crisis 24
neuromuscular junction (NMJ) 13–18

ocular MG 18, 23–4, 34, 35, 37
patholophysiology 13–18, 21
pediatric MG 9, 24
plasmapheresis 28
post-intervention status 39–40
prevalence 7–8
ptosis 18, 23–4, 34, 35, 37
pyridostigmine 19, 26

quality of life score 36, 38
quantitative MG score 33, 34
remission 39
respiratory symptoms 24

severity of MG 19–20, 33, 35
see also treatment-refractory MG
sex 8–10
speech difficulties 24, 34, 35, 37
steroids 10, 26–8
swallowing 34, 35, 37
symptoms 23–4
clinical rating instruments 33–40

thymus gland 18, 28
treatment *see* management
treatment-refractory MG
definition 7
epidemiology 8, 8–10
monitoring 40–1
MuSK Abs 10, 17–18
treatments 19, 29, 41, 42

Notes

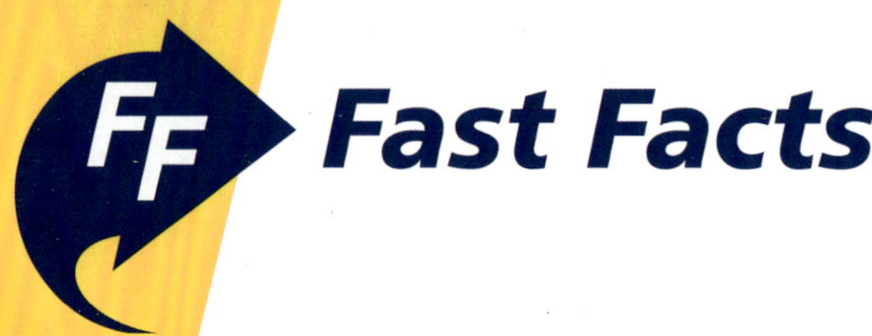

Reading for results

(and tests worth taking)

With so much to read these days, you need to be selective ...

Was this Fast Facts well worth reading?

Has it helped you make good health decisions?

Did it trigger new ideas you'd like to explore?

If so, please post them in the comments box on the relevant page on **www.fastfacts.com**, and check out fellow readers' insights while you're there.

This is also the place to leave questions for the authors' consideration, and to spend 10 minutes on the free **FastTest** to ensure those key points really sunk in, and that you are set to apply them – **result!**

fastfacts.com